HOW TO GET RID OF WEIGHT

Best way to to get rid of your weight very fast

Table of content

HOW TO LOSE WEIGHT

HOW TO LOSE WEIGHT FAST WITHOUT PILLS

HOW TO LOSE WEIGHT FAST

HOW TO LOSE WEIGHT FAST AND EASY

HOW TO LOSE WEIGHT.

You need to drop pounds, presently. What's more, you believe that should do it securely. In any case, how?

To begin with, remember that numerous specialists say all that needs to be said to step by step get thinner. It's bound to remain off. Assuming that you shed pounds excessively quick, you'll lose muscle, bone, and water rather than fat says the Institute of Sustenance and Dietetics.

The foundation's recommendation: Intend to shed 1-2 pounds each week, and stay away from craze diets or items that make guarantees that sound unrealistic. It's ideal to put together your weight reduction concerning transforms you can stay with after some time.

For quicker results, you'll have to work with a specialist, to ensure that you stay sound and get the supplements that you want.

Make an Arrangement

You've presumably heard the expression, "calories in, calories out"; as in, you simply have to consume a greater number of calories than you eat and drink.

Yet, it is quite difficult, as many individuals can tell you from their insight.

Your digestion - - how well your body transforms calories into fuel - - likewise matters. Furthermore, on the off chance that you cut an excessive number of calories, it's awful for you. You delayed your digestion, and that can make you miss the mark on certain supplements.

There are numerous ways you can do this, without cutting calories to an extreme. You could:

Scale back segments.

Sort out the number of calories you get in a typical day, and trim back a little.

Peruse food names to know the number of calories that are in each serving.

Hydrate, so you're not all that hungry.

Anything that technique you use, you'll have to incline toward really great-for-you food varieties like vegetables, natural products, entire grains, and lean protein so you keep up great sustenance. Working with a dietitian is smart, so you make an arrangement that covers those necessities.

Get Responsibility and Backing

Numerous applications can assist you with following your eating. Since you presumably have your cell phone with you constantly, you can utilize it to stay aware of your arrangement. Or on the other hand, keep a pen-and-paper food diary of what you ate and when.

You'll likewise need to have individuals on your side to assist you with remaining spurred and applauding you. So ask your loved ones to help your endeavor to get more fit.

You could likewise need to join a weight reduction bunch where you can discuss how it's going with individuals who can relate. Or on the other hand talk with somebody, you know who's soundly shed pounds. Their consolation is "infectious," positively!

Figure out What Drives You to Eat

At the most essential level, food is fuel. It gives you the energy to get things done. Yet, not many individuals eat only hence. It's at each party. Furthermore, it's where a great deal of us go when we have a harsh day.

You'll have to understand what compels you to need to eat when you're not eager and have an arrangement for those minutes.

The initial step is figuring out what your triggers are. Is it stress, outrage, uneasiness, or wretchedness in a specific piece of your life? Or then again is food your fundamental award when something great occurs?

Then, attempt to see when those sentiments come up and have an arrangement prepared to accomplish something different as opposed to eating. Might you at some point go for a stroll? Text a companion?

In conclusion, reward yourself for settling on an alternate decision. Simply don't involve food as the award.

Reset What and When You Eat

You don't need to go vegetarian, without gluten, or quit a specific nutrition class to get in shape. You're bound to keep the pounds off for good if it's something you can live with as long as possible.

In any case, it appears to be legit to chop way down on, or completely cut out, void calories.

Limit added sugars. These are the sugars in treats, cakes, sugar-improved drinks, and different things - - not the sugars that are normally in organic products, for example. Sweet food varieties frequently have a lot of calories however a couple of supplements. Intend to spend under 10% of your everyday calories on added sugars.

Be finicky about carbs. You can conclude which ones you eat, and how much. Search for those that are falling short on the glycemic record (for example, asparagus is lower on the glycemic file than a potato) or lower in carbs per serving than others. Entire grains are preferred decisions over handled things since handling eliminates key supplements like fiber, iron, and B nutrients. They might be added back, for example, in "advanced" bread.

Incorporate protein. It's wonderful and will assist with keeping up your muscles. There are a veggie lovers and vegetarian sources (nuts, beans, and soy are a couple), as well as lean meat, poultry, fish, and dairy.

Most Americans get sufficient protein however could decide to get it from more streamlined sources, so you may as of now have a lot in your eating regimen. Your accurate protein needs rely upon your age, orientation, and how dynamic you are.

Warm up to great fats. Modest quantities of fat can help you feel full and less like you're on a careful nutritional plan. The better decisions are those in fish, nuts and seeds, and olive oil. Those have unsaturated fats - - polyunsaturated or monounsaturated fats, explicitly.

Top off on fiber. You can get that from vegetables, entire grains, natural products - - any plant food will have fiber. Some have more than others. Top sources incorporate artichokes, green peas, broccoli, lentils, and lima beans. Among natural products, raspberries lead the rundown.

Eat on a more regular basis. If you eat 5-6 times each day, it could keep hunger under control. You could divide your calories

similarly across those scaled-down dinners, or make some greater than others. You should design partitions with the goal that you don't wind up eating beyond anything you could have expected.
And Dinner Substitutions? These items will control your calories. They're helpful and remove the mystery of eating less junk food. Once more, however, you'll have to change your dietary patterns to keep the load off assuming that you go off the dinner substitutions.
Watch your beverages. One simple method for getting in shape rapidly is to remove fluid calories, like pop, and juice. Supplant them with zero-calorie drinks like lemon water, unsweetened tea, or dark coffee.
Diet beverages will save you calories, contrasted, and sweet refreshments. In any case, on the off chance that you, go after a treat or other treat since you're as yet eager or you assume you saved an adequate number of calories for it, that plan misfires.

Would it be a good idea for you to Quick?
You could imagine that fasting is a speedy method for dropping pounds. Yet, it's smarter to have an eating plan that you can adhere to over the long run and that squeezes into your way of life.
More examination is had to be aware assuming that fasting is protected long haul. Most investigations of the impacts of irregular fasting have been finished on overweight, moderately-aged grown-ups. More examination is expected to decide whether ok for individuals who are more seasoned or more youthful or individuals at a solid weight.

All diets aren't something similar. Some include skirting all food. There are likewise diets where you eat every other day. There hasn't been a great deal of examination on how well now and again fasting functions over the long haul.

During the principal days of your quick, you might feel eager and cranky. You may likewise get obstructed. Also, you will not have the energy to do a lot, truly. Hydrate and take a day-to-day multivitamin. You ought to likewise tell your primary care physician, particularly assuming you take meds that will presumably be changed.

Recollect that assuming you do quick, you'll in any case have to change your dietary patterns once your quick closures.

Regardless of how you launch your weight reduction, the most ideal way to keep it off is with dependable way of life changes, similar to a good dieting plan and active work. On the off chance that you don't know where to begin, the number of calories to cut, or how to do it securely, you should counsel an enrolled dietitian.

HOW TO LOSE WEIGHT FAST WITHOUT PILLS

Anorexics might lose as much as 15 to 20 pounds each month, agreeing your weight. How much weight reduction is reliant upon the individual's body type, how much activity he gets, and his by and large dietary admission.

At the point when a body is famished of its supplements, practice becomes more enthusiastically, Orgclinic.com proceeds to make sense of it. Likewise, when a body is famished, it goes to utilizing its muscle tissue and muscle versus fat for supplements. Anorexics lose muscle definition because the body needs to consume itself to get by. As the body consumes the muscle versus fat and muscle tissue, weight reduction eases back, and body closure may ultimately happen.

The speed of weight reduction relies upon the specific strategies utilized by the singular anorexic, as indicated by Orgclinic.com. Individuals with anorexia nervosa utilize different measures to radically lessen food admission like cleansing, taking diuretics, and not eating.

Anorexics likewise will generally practice unreasonably, says the Workplace on Lady's Wellbeing, a part of the U.S. Branch of Wellbeing and Human Administrations. The body answers these activities by dialing the digestion and crushing the spirit of the muscle tissues, among other framework changes.

Anorexia is a dietary problem that can be deadly, as per the Workplace on Ladies' Wellbeing, yet anorexics can get better with direction from specialists, nutritionists, and advisors.

HOW TO LOSE WEIGHT FAST

Numerous understudies need to manage new everyday environments and equilibrium a strong class load, all while making new companions and attempting to keep a public activity.

Dietary patterns likewise will more often than not change in school. Late evenings out, incessant liquor admission and restricted quality food choices can negatively affect your general well-being.

These variables can prompt weight gain and other medical problems over the long run.

While numerous undergrads go to craze eat less and other unfortunate and unreasonable techniques to get thinner rapidly, these can wind up causing more damage than great over the long haul.

Notwithstanding, it's feasible to reach and keep a sound body weight during school. A couple of key changes won't just assist with working on your dietary decisions yet, in addition, upgrade your general mental and actual well-being.

This article investigates how to reach and keep a solid body weight during school, in addition to a couple of tips on the most proficient method to improve your general prosperity.

Share on Pinterest

Why is weight gain in school so normal?

Concentrates on the show that most understudies put on weight, particularly during their most memorable year.

A 2015 survey of 32 examinations found that over 60% of undergrads put on weight during their first year. (All things considered (1

The survey likewise found that understudies put on weight at a lot quicker rate than everybody.

This isn't shocking given that undergrads can have altogether unexpected ways of life in comparison to individuals who are not in school.

What causes school weight gain?

Changes in dietary patterns can altogether add to weight gain during school.

Research shows that undergrads will generally eat less nutritious food varieties, like eggs and vegetables, and all the more exceptionally handled and sweet things, like doughnuts and seared food varieties. In addition, understudies will generally drink more liquor, which can prompt weight gain.

Be that as it may, there are likewise different variables to consider.

For instance, most understudies are under a lot of pressure.

They might be encountering strain to prevail in classes, the monetary weight of educational loans, and the trouble of adjusting scholarly and public activity. Stress is emphatically connected with weight gain.

Notwithstanding stress, some understudies experience misery and tension, which are additionally connected to weight gain.

Understudies similarly will generally be less dynamic and get less rest than the typical individual, the two of which are propensities that can add to weight gain and adversely influence by and large wellbeing

As may be obvious, many variables add to weight gain during school.

Consequently, you can't treat the issue with dietary changes alone. Rather, a comprehensive way to deal with diet, way of life, and mental prosperity are significantly more compelling for keeping a solid load all through school and then some.

It's likewise critical to take note that during your late teenage and mid-20s, body changes are typical. Your body might change shape and size as you proceed to develop and create.

Might it at any point influence long-haul well-being?

While the time you spend at school just includes a little part of your life, how you treat your body during this time can influence your well-being as you age.

Concentrates on the show that individuals who are overweight in their teenagers and 20s are bound to be overweight as they become older. In addition, weight gain during early adulthood is related to persistent ailments sometime down the road

For instance, a recent report that included 7,289 grown-ups observed that individuals who were overweight during early adulthood were fundamentally bound to foster diabetes further down the road

Studies have likewise found a connection between juvenile stoutness and a more serious gamble of stroke, hypertension, and coronary vein sickness, the most widely recognized kind of coronary illness

Even though your decisions during youthful adulthood might just impact your well-being further down the road, it's basic to comprehend that you can improve your well-being.

Caring more for yourself doesn't imply that your eating routine and way of life decisions must be great. It implies tracking down a well-thought-out plan that works for you — and that you can keep up with the long haul.

Sound ways of getting thinner in school

Eating restoratively is only one piece of the riddle concerning keeping a sound load in school.

Here are vital ways of getting thinner securely and further developing your general well-being when you're in school.

Eat nutritious food varieties on a more regular basis and unhealthy foods on rare occasions

Craze slims down and centers around hardship and limitation. Staying away from them is ideal.

They don't work for long-haul weight reduction, and they can prompt critical emotional well-being issues and the advancement of an undesirable relationship with food (15

All things being equal, foster an eating design that turns out best for your body by zeroing in on entire, supplement-thick food varieties like vegetables, natural products, vegetables, protein sources (e.g., eggs and chicken), and solid fats (e.g., nuts and olive oil).

Attempt to scale back food sources and drinks that are firmly connected to weight gain. These incorporate sugar-improved refreshments like pop and caffeinated drinks, cheap food, improved heated products, and refined carbs like sweet breakfast oats (16

For instance, on the off chance that you're accustomed to eating a huge bowl of sweet oat and a cup of squeezed orange in the feasting corridor every morning, have a go at deciding on a bowl of plain oats finished off with nuts or seeds, new natural product, and a dab of Greek yogurt all things being equal.

Try to routinely fuel your body. Try not to skip dinners to get in shape. Your smartest choice is to pay attention to your body and eat when you're ravenous.

If you don't know where to begin, verify whether your school offers dietary directing through understudy well-being administrations.

Find exercises you love

Generally, undergrads who are attempting to lose an abundance of muscle versus fat join exercise centers and partake in tiresome exercise classes. Albeit working out can advance weight reduction, it's not quite as significant as being genuinely dynamic consistently.

If you appreciate going to the exercise center, going to exercise classes and making your exercises might be a decent decision for you.

Be that as it may, on the off chance that you're not an exercise center individual or feel awkward working out before others, it's feasible to keep a solid weight and even get in shape while never swinging by a wellness place.

The following are a couple of ways of remaining dynamic in school without going to the exercise center:

Stroll to your classes.

Go for a run outside.

Climb with companions in a neighborhood park or backwoods.

Take a dip at the school pool.

Evaluate a YouTube exercise class in your apartment.

Getting a stage tracker can assist you with surveying how dynamic you are and assist you with gradually expanding your movement levels. For instance, assuming you're as of now averaging 3,000 stages each day, have a go at adding 1,000 moves toward that.

When you're reliably arriving at that objective, add one more 1,000 stages until you're arriving at something like 7,500 stages each day, which specialists consider "dynamic" (19

Concentrates on the show that arriving at least 10,000 stages each day can support weight reduction and work on physical and psychological well-being (20

Oversee pressure

Stress can adversely influence your body weight and negatively affect your psychological wellness (3

Figuring out how to deal with your feelings of anxiety is significant to your general prosperity. Finding outlets that assist with easing pressure in your youngsters and mid-twenties can assist with setting a solid starting point for future pressure on the executives.

It might require some investment, and you could find that what works for others doesn't be guaranteed to assist with alleviating pressure for you. To that end, it's critical to evaluate various pressure the board practices to see what works.

Here are a few exercises that might assist with easing pressure (21

yoga

contemplation

taking part in actual work

investing energy outside climbing or strolling

paying attention to or making music

Breathing activity

investing energy with friends and family

On the off chance that you want assistance dealing with your feelings of anxiety, working with a psychological well-being instructor can help. Guiding administrations are accessible at most schools.

Get sufficient rest

Rest is basic to by and large well-being. Not getting enough of it has been reliably connected to weight gain in research studies (9

Appreciating late-night home bases with friends is alive and well and ordinary. Be that as it may, on most evenings of the week, ensure you get the Public Rest Establishment's base for youthful grown-ups: 7 hours of rest. This will assist you with keeping a solid weight

Restricting screen time and making a relieving, dim climate in your room can help you fall and stay unconscious.

Treat any hidden clinical issues

A few medical issues related to weight gain might create during your late teenagers and mid-20s.

For instance, polycystic ovary syndrome(PCOS) and Hashimoto's hypothyroidism can appear during puberty and youthful adulthood

Clinical sorrow, which is additionally connected with weight gain, is normal among school mature individuals

Assuming you have encountered fast, unexplained weight gain or are encountering different side effects that are influencing your well-being, it means quite a bit to visit your medical services supplier to preclude any possible fundamental ailments.

Furthermore, dietary problems are normal among school mature individuals. These incorporate anorexia, bulimia, and voraciously consuming food issues (BED). These are serious ailments that should be treated by a certified medical care supplier.

On the off chance that you figure you might have a dietary issue, contact a medical care supplier or somebody you trust to seek the therapy you want.

Diminish your liquor utilization

Concentrates on demonstrating the way that weighty drinking during school can prompt weight gain.

For instance, a review that remembered information from 7,941 youthful grown-ups observed that successive weighty drinking was related to a 41% higher gamble of being overweight and a 36% higher gamble of creating stoutness 5 years after the fact (28

In addition, drinking an excess of liquor isn't great for your general well-being and can prompt side effects of despondency and nervousness

Even though liquor can be essential for your school insight, making protected, sound bound is significant,

HOW TO LOSE WEIGHT FAST AND EASY

Concerning counting calories, there are many ways of thinking. Certain individuals put stock in removing carbs totally, while others depend on irregular fasting. In all actuality, practically any change you make to your ongoing eating regimen will assist with working on your well-being and prosperity.

Clean eating, by definition, is eating entire or natural food varieties. It's truly not convoluted, however, it requires some work and arranging. It doesn't expect you to count carbs, sugar, calories, or macros. It's anything but an eating routine. It's a way of life change (Assuming you're feigning exacerbation at that pondering how frequently you've heard that, stay with me!).

Clean eating, as I would like to think, is the ideal "beginning stage" for getting into the propensity for practicing good eating habits. It's a basic and achievable way of life change. The issue with vogue eating fewer carbs is they are exceptionally difficult to keep up long haul (or they request excessively, excessively quick). Who needs to count macros until the end of their life, or net carbs, or be denied an apple? Who needs to feel coerced for eating a dry piece of newly prepared sourdough bread? Nobody!

Clean eating permits you to partake in the food varieties you love, with, I concede, somewhat more exertion on the cooking front without feeling a very way. How incredible is that? While you're attempting to sort out some way to begin eating solid as a novice, there's truly not much to sort out. If it is handled, it arrives in a container or bundle bound with additives and synthetic compounds, search for another option, and you're coming.

Why We Hunger for Low-quality Food Over Good Food

Unhealthy food is effectively open and reasonable. It's not difficult to go through a drive-through or get something undesirable at the supermarket since it's all over. The accommodation factor is genuine. Contrast that with attempting to discover a few new natural products or vegetables, and you'll understand.

Not exclusively is unhealthy food more available, but at the same time, it's designed to be habit-forming. Food sources like chips, treats, and candy are intended to hit the appropriate buttons in our minds, they're pungent, sweet, crunchy, and smooth! Organizations include synthetic compounds and different fixings to keep you needing more (i.e., filling their pockets!). At the point when you eat low-quality food, your cerebrum discharges dopamine which is the reason we will generally desire it over better choices.

Different variables, similar to candida (yeast), can assume control over your stomach's well-being, conveying messages to your cerebrum that then, at that point, advise you to take care of its sugar. Many individuals mark down stomach well-being and a candida excess as babble, yet it is perhaps of the most controlling microscopic organisms and might be at fault for your sugar desires.

Many individuals laugh at the possibility that your stomach has some control over your feelings and, surprisingly, emotional wellness. If you will generally experience the ill effects of discouragement, nervousness, or something like that, it might be in every way connected back to the mind's stomach hub. Many examinations have started to spring up lately, confirming this, even though it very well might be difficult to stomach the thought (in all seriousness!)

It very well may be hard to bring an end to vices and desires, yet entirely it's most certainly not feasible. With a smidgen of exertion, you can retrain your mind and mend your stomach to want quality food sources over horrible ones!

10 Good dieting Tips On the most proficient method to begin eating smart for fledglings

The primary genuine move toward practicing good eating habits is understanding that there's no need to focus on denying yourself the relative multitude of food varieties you love. It's tied in with finding harmony between gobbling what you appreciate and stepping up certain propensities so your eating regimen turns out to be more adjusted such that works for you.

You'll see that a considerable lot of these warns cross over and play off one another! Play with those that reverberate and leave the rest. At last, smart dieting appears to be somewhat unique for everybody, and the way to find a practice change is to track down the methodology that works for you, your body, and your way of life.

YOU CAN Pay attention TO Every one of the TEN Smart dieting TIPS IN THIS VIDEO!

Good dieting Tip #1: BE simple, delicate, and inquisitive with yourself

I know a large number of you believe I should bounce directly into the activity steps, and I get it, Yet we need to recall that for us to make positive changes in our lives, we need to come from a positive profound state. This is fundamental for novices to truly accept as it's the establishment of your relationship with food pushing ahead. So many of us have gained from the media and the eating regimen industry that eating better or getting more fit must be hard, and we need to push and limit and deny our direction to the end goal, However obviously, that doesn't work.

At the point when you are continually pushing and reprimanding yourself - you make a lot of pessimistic inclinations, and it's truly challenging it is certainly feasible, to make a positive change from a pessimistic profound state. So focus on a kinder way. Advise yourself that stage one is to be, simple kind, and inquisitive with yourself so you can make changes that will work for yourself as well as your way of life reasonably and feasibly.

Smart dieting Tip #2 Spotlight on Genuine Entire Food varieties (otherwise known as Perfect Eating)

The absolute most significant shift anybody can make with their eating is to start to zero in on eating Genuine, entire food varieties as near their normal state as could be expected, more often than not. These are food varieties that come from the earth as well as creatures assuming you eat creature items.

These are the food sources that your grandma would eat - they are straightforward food sources and they are scrumptious. Think veggies, organic products, sound normal fats like avocados, nuts, and seeds, quality proteins like fish, fed meats, lentils, and great quality entire grains; like wild rice, cereal, and quinoa. While this is a straightforward shift, it is a significant shift! I would contend that is the absolute most significant shift you can make with regard to good dieting as a novice.

Good dieting Tip #3: Stay away from Exceptionally Handled Food sources

Falling off of the impact points of zeroing in on genuine entire food varieties, we truly need to keep away from or limit profoundly handled food sources. Profoundly handled food sources are food-like substances that are made in processing plants and made to energize your tastebuds yet not to sustain your body. Removing handled food sources is, indeed, quite possibly the hardest thing to do while you're beginning your smart dieting venture.

There are various kinds of handled food sources. For instance, oats is a softly handled food, as is grown bread or frozen veggie veggies. In any case, these are not the handled food varieties I would stress over. The handled food varieties I'm alluding to are the Exceptionally handled food sources, they aren't food by any stretch of the imagination, and in some way or another figure out how to fill most of the racks at the supermarket.

These are food-like substances that are healthfully void, meaning they offer no health benefit and are extremely sub-par concerning feeling sustained and fulfilled by your dinner. These are food sources that come in bundles and keep going on racks for quite a long time.

Some could contend that these food-like items taste great (since they are stacked with salt, sugar, and bad quality oils and are intended to energize your taste buds), yet past flavor - they don't offer anything of real value and are famous for screwing with chemicals, glucose, and stomach wellbeing. So essentially searching for less handled to all the more entire food choices can take your good dieting game to an unheard-of level. On the off chance that you can't peruse or grasp fixings on a mark, rack it!

Smart dieting Tip #4 Associate With Your Appetite

Intermittently when we are attempting to eat better, we focus on outside data to let us know what and when to eat. This is the very thing that winds up hindering and eventually prompting the end of most amateurs' efforts to begin and keep up with intelligent dieting propensities. The issue with this is that it makes the deception that you can't confide in your body and consequently separates us from our regular craving signals. So the basic practice here is to exit your brain, overlook the food rules and mental plans, and drop once more into your body.

An incredible method for working on dropping once more into the body and out of the mind is to pose two basic inquiries. Before eating - ask yourself, "Am I hungry?" And when part of the way through your feast, stop and ask your body, "Have I had enough?".

This can take some training on the off chance that you have been eating as indicated by the clock or the outside food rules - Yet - whenever we discover some new information, we want to effortlessly ourselves the space to rehearse. So let it feel uneven as you start to reconnect to your body and trust that your body is sufficiently insightful to be aware.

Good dieting Tip #5: Examination with your Macronutrient Equilibrium

We as a whole hear a great deal about macronutrients nowadays, and keeping in mind that I am not proposing that you count and work out your macronutrients, I do believe it's essential to consider the equilibrium of carbs, proteins, and fats you have with every dinner.

On the off chance that you will generally have a starch-weighty eating regimen, essentially including proteins and sound fats with your dinners can truly assist you with feeling fulfilled and satisfied after you're finished eating, which can likewise decide when and what you need to eat straight away.

Does this mean you can never eat a plate of flapjacks or a bowl of pasta? Not really - Yet assuming that you are somebody who battles with weight, indulging, or you essentially observe that you're not fulfilled after a feast, or that you are eager soon after eating dinner - playing with your macronutrient equilibrium can be a truly incredible spot to try.

Take a stab at beginning your day with a dinner wealthy in protein and solid fats, and simply notice to perceive how this feels for yourself as well as your body. This could be a veggie omelet with a few cheddar, a bowl of natural full-fat greek yogurt with nuts seeds, and berries, or some almond flour hotcakes. The situation is to play and notice! See what feels best for yourself as well as your body.

Good dieting Tip #6: Quality Over Calories

Certain individuals instruct that a calorie is a calorie, and it doesn't make any difference what you eat as long as you don't eat a bigger number of

calories than you want. I for one think this is a shallow and misrepresented way to deal with

www.ingramcontent.com/pod-product-compliance
Lightning Source LLC
LaVergne TN
LVHW020543160826
845677LV00015B/4177

* 9 7 9 8 3 5 6 6 0 6 5 1 9 *